CANDLE MAGIC
JOURNAL AND HANDBOOK

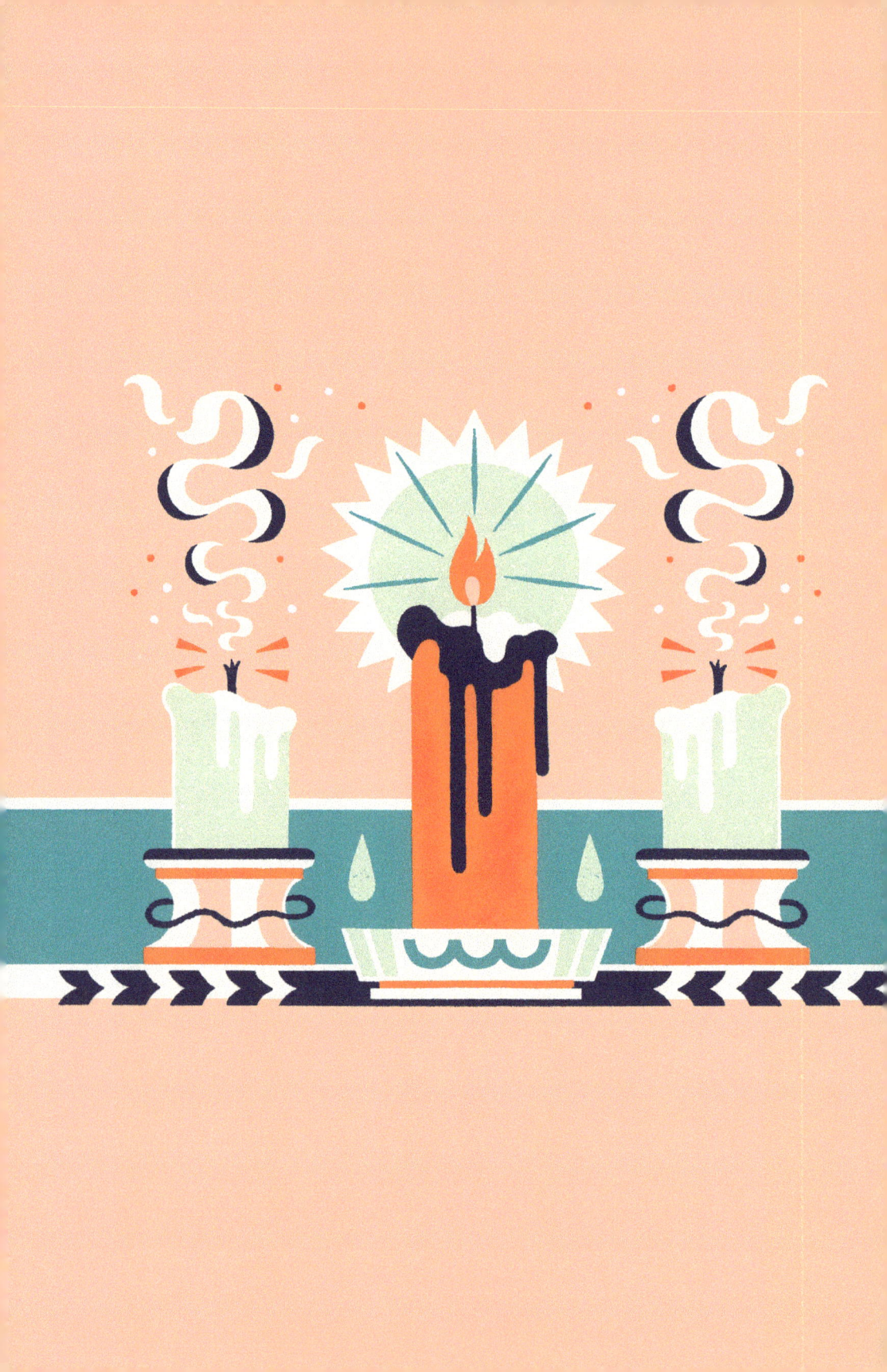

CANDLE MAGIC
JOURNAL
AND HANDBOOK

A Guide to Performing Spells, Setting Intentions,
and Recording Your Magical Practice

PATTI WIGINGTON

ROCKRIDGE
PRESS

Interior and Cover Designer: Lindsey Dekker
Art Producer: Janice Ackerman
Editor: Brian Sweeting
Production Manager: Holly Haydash
Production Editor: Cassie Gitkin

Paperback ISBN: 978-1-63878-422-7
eBook ISBN: 978-1-63878-787-7
R0

THIS BOOK IS FOR ALICE,
WHO BROUGHT THE LIGHT
OF A THOUSAND CANDLES
INTO MY LIFE.

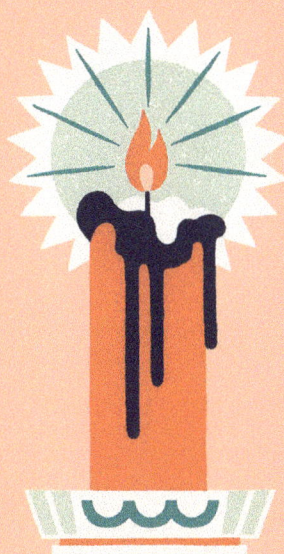

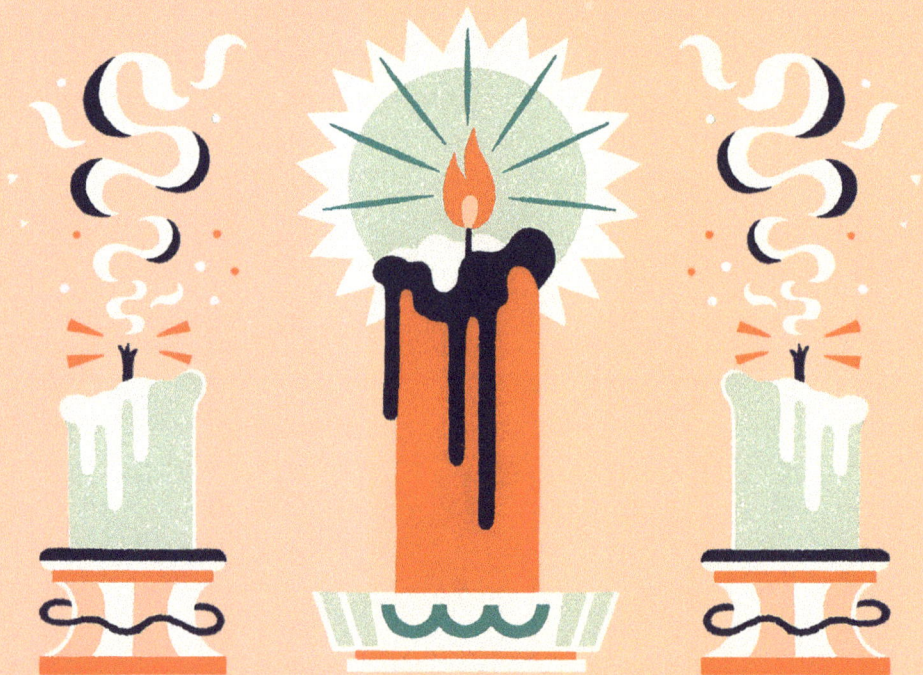

CONTENTS

INTRODUCTION

When I first began practicing as a witch and pagan, more than three decades ago, I was young and financially struggling. There were so many things in the witchcraft books I wanted to buy! Fancy athames, beautiful crystals, heavy cast-iron cauldrons, exotic herbs—you name it, I couldn't afford it. But I discovered pretty quickly that one thing I *could* work into my budget—even if it meant rolling quarters to go to the laundromat—was a box of candles.

There was a tiny corner store not far from my apartment, and I visited frequently to buy little votive candles in every color imaginable—they were three for a dollar! For just a few bucks, I'd have a dozen candles in hand and could make any sort of magic I wished. Since that time, I've expanded my use of tools—eventually including those herbs, crystals, and other goodies—but candle magic was my first foray into spellwork, and it's still a cornerstone of my magic.

There's something so raw, almost primal, about staring into the flame of a candle, watching it burn. Fire both creates and destroys, and even the tiniest flame can be mighty. There is power in it, and yet it's deceptively simple to work with. In many magical traditions today, candle magic is considered one of the most basic forms of spellwork; as such, it's a great place for beginners to start learning to practice. Because it's so effective, however, it's also a type of magic you'll see many veteran practitioners engaging in. No matter where you fall on that spectrum, it's my hope that you'll use this handbook as a way to learn more about the transformational power of candle magic and how you can use it to bring about change in your own life.

As you meander through the pages of this book, you may encounter spell ingredients that you don't have readily available. If that happens, don't worry! Consider this handbook a template and use the basic concepts within it as the foundation to create your own spells from scratch. It's much like the old adage about giving someone a fish. You can eat for a day if you're given a fish, but if someone shows you *how* to catch a fish—well, you can eat for a really long time.

Also, remember this book is not intended to be a comprehensive manifesto on candle magic (although there is a detailed list of some really awesome resources to check out at the back). Instead, think of it as a guide that will help you put creative and critical thought into your magic and help you understand not just what to do but *why* to do it. Successful magic consists of several important elements, including intention, purpose, and work. Candles are simply a tool to help you achieve your goals—but you'll still have to set your intention, determine your purpose, and do the work to manifest change.

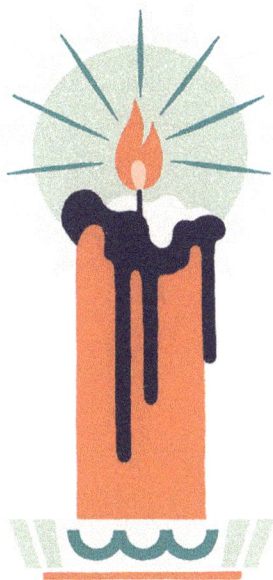

HOW TO USE THIS BOOK

What can you expect in this book? As mentioned, it's not a Candle Magic 101 class—although we'll start off in part 1 with a brief overview of things you should know. You can view that as a refresher if you've worked with candle magic before. If you're new to this type of spellwork, see that section as a list of things into which you may want to take a deep dive. In part 2, you'll find a series of journal prompts that will help you do a bit of self-reflection and introspection. The better you know yourself, the better you'll be able to focus your magic and set your goals. Finally, in part 3, there is a collection of candle spells for a variety of purposes, as well as blank spaces for you to record your own spellwork and evaluate the outcomes and results. It's important to note that most people in the magical community avoid magic that deliberately harms others. All the spells in this book are designed to manifest transformation that benefits the self in a healthy and positive way.

Although working through this handbook in order is certainly encouraged, if you feel called to jump around and do things in a different order, go for it! Write in the pages. Dog-ear the corners. Doodle in the margins. Do everything you need to make it feel like your own and make it truly magical.

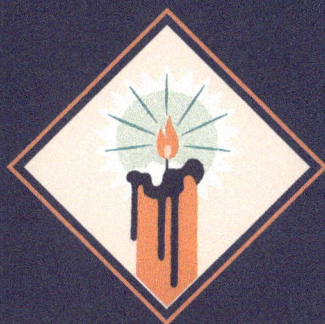

CANDLE SAFETY

Candles—especially those used in magic—should bring comfort and joy and inspire relaxation and creativity. However, that doesn't mean you should ignore common sense. You should follow some basic safety tips when doing candle magic. Always burn your candle on a flat, heat-resistant surface, far from any flammable materials. Use a candle holder, a fire-safe plate or cauldron, or a dish of sand or soil to hold it in place. Be sure to remove any decorative items, such as flammable tags or charms, from the candle before lighting it.

Don't leave a lit candle unattended; if you need to stop in the middle of a magical working, extinguish the candle. You can always relight it later, but you can't unburn your home. Finally, be sure to keep candles away from children and inquisitive pets. Remember, it can take mere seconds for a beautiful ritual to become a dire emergency.

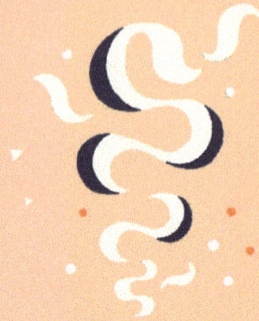

INTENTION IS ONE WITH CAUSE AND EFFECT. INTENTION DETERMINES OUTCOME. AND IF YOU'RE STUCK AND NOT MOVING FORWARD, YOU HAVE TO CHECK THE THOUGHT AND ACTION THAT CREATED THE CIRCUMSTANCE.

—OPRAH WINFREY

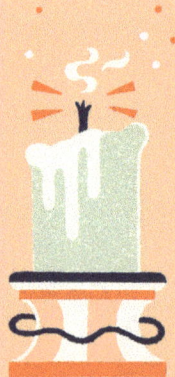

PART 1

A BRIEF GUIDE TO CANDLE MAGIC

Although this book isn't designed to be an exhaustive manual on how to practice candle magic, there are certainly a few things you'll want to keep in mind as you dive deeper into your practice. In this section, we'll be talking about the history of fire throughout human existence: How did a source of light and heat become associated with magic? What's so special about candles anyway?

We'll also review some of the basics of candle magic practice, including the symbolism—or correspondences—of the various colors you may want to select for your workings. You'll learn about the different types of candles and why you might choose one variety over another. In addition, we'll discuss how to prepare your candles for magical use, including cleansing and consecration. You'll also learn some key components of setting your intentions and turning your magic into something active, rather than just "wish-craft."

FIRE: AN OLD POWER

Fire is one of the four classical elements found in many of today's magical traditions—the other three are earth, air, and water. Associated with strong will and energy, fire can both create and destroy. The earliest evidence of humankind's control of fire—dating back about 1.7 million years—was found in South Africa's Wonderwerk Cave. Early people used it to make tools, stay warm at night, and frighten away predators. Caves in Israel show evidence that some 300,000 to 400,000 years ago, their inhabitants were regularly roasting meat. Once humans learned how to deliberately start, maintain, and move a fire, they were able to control and expand their diet, and the cooking hearth itself likely formed a social center of the community.

As communities formed, so too did structured spiritual practice. Fire brought us not only physical light but also spiritual illumination. Fire appears in the myth and folklore of cultures around the world, usually in the context of both destruction and creation. It is often represented as a living entity that needs nourishment and tending to thrive; like people, without those things it fades and dies. In many religious practices, fire is seen as the holiest of the four elements. It is never tainted or polluted, and it frequently represents eternal life, the universal symbol of the Divine.

Fire is, in a spiritual sense, the ultimate purifier, consuming everything in its path and changing matter from one form to another. In many belief systems today, fire remains the bridge between the physical realm and that of the sacred, a connector from our mundane world to the dominion of the spiritual.

THE POWER OF CANDLES

Perhaps the most valuable human discovery is that we can control fire and bring it into our homes and places of worship. The ancient Egyptians dipped reeds in rendered fat, creating the first candles, and the Romans took the process a step further by incorporating the wick into candle construction. Later, European candle makers learned that beeswax candles burned more cleanly than those made from tallow, and during America's colonial period, whale oil was crystallized into a hard wax, creating an even brighter light than beeswax. In the 19th century, paraffin was introduced, leading to the mass production of machine-fabricated candles.

Candles have been used to light homes and churches, as part of rituals and ceremonies, and even as a way of marking time. Nearly every civilization has employed some form of candle in important religious ceremonies; go into any church, synagogue, or temple, and you're likely to see candles burning. They are lit to honor the Divine, show respect for the dead, and create an illuminated path between our world and the next. When we use candles in transformative magic, we are carrying on an age-old tradition.

THE BASICS OF CANDLE MAGIC

Candles represent all four of the classical elements, which are often highly important to practitioners of modern witchcraft, combined into one convenient package. The solid wax of a fresh, unused candle is reminiscent of the stable, firm grounding of the earth. Air, the soft breeze of inspiration, fans the flame and allows magic to build. There is the flame itself, the fire, which both destroys and creates, and steers our energies and passions. Finally, as the wax melts into liquid, one can't help but be reminded of the gentle, cleansing flow of water.

Today, we who practice witchcraft and other spiritual traditions often incorporate candles into our rites and rituals. Candles are the foundation of the simplest type of spellwork; if you have one, you can cast a spell by a number of different methods. One of the easiest ways to use a candle in magic is to inscribe your intentions into the wax. You may also choose to dress it in magical oils and herbs that correspond with your goals and purpose, or simply burn it to send your intentions out into the universe. Many people use candles for divination as well; fire scrying is a popular method in which the practitioner stares into the flame to look for images and symbols. You can also seek out messages by dripping the candle's melted wax into a bowl of cold water and then interpreting the shapes.

As an added bonus, candles aren't usually costly; you can typically obtain them inexpensively and make magic within your budget. It's a good idea to keep a few candles on hand in a variety of colors and sizes, but don't go too far overboard; as your practice develops, you may find you prefer working with specific types. Don't waste money on candles you'll never use.

ADDING ADDITIONAL INGREDIENTS TO YOUR PRACTICE

You may want to add other ingredients into your candle magic workings, and we'll go into more detail on ways to do so in the coming sections. Using oils or herbs can help give your magic a boost and enhance the way your spell performs.

If you're adding bits and pieces to a candle, keep safety in mind. With jar candles, be extra cautious. Don't add crystals or stones onto the top, as they can create excessive heat and cause the jar to shatter. Avoid pressing glitter, coffee beans, and other flammable items into the top of the wax. Oils and dried herbs should never be placed too close to the wick; keep them around the sides of the candle, and use them in moderation.

You can dress your candle in a variety of ways, but most people find it easiest to apply a thin coat of light unscented oil with a brush or a piece of cotton. Brush the oil toward you for attraction and spells intended to draw things to you, or away from you for workings that banish and eliminate. Once you've coated the candle with oil, roll it in a powdered herb mixture, or simply take a pinch of your dried herbs and sprinkle them lightly over the oil.

COLORS AND THEIR POWERS

The use of color correspondences in magic not only is cost-effective but also makes sense. Each color contains its own unique energy, and you can draw on that power to manifest change. By combining the symbolism of colors with candle magic basics, it's possible to create a spell for just about anything. The magic of a color doesn't have to come only from a candle; consider adding flowers, fabric, ribbons, or even colored paper into your workings.

RED

Use red for spellwork connected to passion and energy or love and seduction, or as a power color when you need a boost. Red, a color of courage and confidence, will give your sex life some extra vitality and can help you stabilize as you prepare for conflict and challenges on the road ahead.

ORANGE

Orange is the color of attraction, encouragement, and creativity. It comes in handy for workings that draw new opportunities, inspire the creative muse, and establish deep, meaningful emotional connections with others. Use orange if you're seeking positivity, fun, and adventure in your life.

YELLOW

It's hard to feel sad when you've got yellow around you! It's a bright, sunny color, tied to protective and persuasive energies. Related to feelings of self-empowerment, yellow helps boost your confidence and self-esteem, allowing you to spread joy—and when you spread joy, those around you will often see things your way.

GREEN

It's probably no surprise that green is a color of financial abundance; use it for workings designed to draw money your way. It's also associated with matters of fertility, although that doesn't necessarily mean physical fertility. What do you want to create, grow, and nurture in your life?

INDIGO

Connected to our intuitive perception, indigo is useful for developing your psychic abilities, shedding emotional baggage, and getting in touch with self-realization. This color is valuable in spellwork designed to heal trauma and come to terms with emotional vulnerability, as well as representing fairness, integrity, and the authentic self.

BLUE

When it comes to healing magic, blue is the perfect addition to your spellwork. It's tied to not only physical well-being but also mental and emotional health. Blue is associated with communication and honesty, so use it for spells related to finding the truth or establishing trust.

PINK

Although red is associated with passionate love, pink is far more platonic. It corresponds with sweet, innocent love, as well as friendship and mutually respectful partnerships. Pink is nurturing and caring whether toward others or yourself. Work with pink for self-care or for helping people in a relationship understand one another on a deeper level.

PURPLE

For many people, purple is a power color. The color of royalty in days gone by, it is related to ambition, success, and being in control of one's situation. It's also deeply tied to our intuition and can be invoked for workings related to the psychic self and connecting with the Divine.

BROWN

Feeling disconnected from the natural world around you? Use brown to bring you closer to the earth and the elements. Brown is also valuable in workings related to animals and is traditionally associated with the stability, security, and grounding presence of home and domestic life.

GRAY

Somewhere on the spectrum between black and white, gray lingers in its many shades. It's a bit mysterious and elegant, and can be useful for workings related to business, wisdom, and a sense of authority. Consider spells involving the color gray when you seek balance, neutrality, and compromise.

BLACK

Contrary to popular opinion, magic involving the color black isn't evil. In fact, black is a powerful color of protection. Use it for workings to keep yourself safe, both physically and emotionally. Black can be used to banish things that no longer serve you or to bind those who might wish to do you harm.

WHITE

Associated with truth and the higher self, white is the color to use when you're looking for knowledge, unity, and a sense of peace. White corresponds to cleansing and purity and is often used in blessings and consecration rituals. In many magical traditions, a white candle is seen as a valid alternative for any other color; when using a white candle as a substitute, focus your intention on your purpose just as you would for the color it is replacing.

SILVER

Silver is the color of the full moon, so it shouldn't be a surprise that it's associated with lunar magic, intuition, and psychic development. Use silver in divination spells, dream magic, scrying, or workings tied to the ocean's ebb and flow.

GOLD

Whereas silver is connected to the moon, gold is the color of the sun and is deeply connected to solar magic, power and energy, and material gain. Use gold for business endeavors, for money magic, or even to bring about a favorable judgment in a court of law.

TYPES AND QUALITIES OF CANDLES

In many cases, you'll find that candle magic spells don't call for a specific type of candle. In these circumstances, what you'll use is entirely up to you. Sometimes, however, there's a meaning behind the recommendation for a certain kind of candle. Everyone's practice is a little different, so if a spell says to use a certain type or size, think about what those reasons could be.

In some magical traditions, unscented candles are always used. Scents can be distracting, and if you have aroma sensitivities, it may be best to use candles without fragrance. There are times when it may be logical to use a scented candle, however: If you're doing a working to help you relax, for instance, a lavender scent will certainly aid you in achieving your goal. If you do choose to use a fragrant candle, make sure the scent is one that aligns with your intent.

Finally, because most practitioners prefer to use a fresh candle for each working, consider burn time when choosing your candle. Put some thought into your selection. For instance, if a working calls for you to light a candle each night for a week, don't pick a tea light; use a larger candle. On the other hand, if the spell is designed to be worked in a single evening, you may want to try a votive or other smaller candle. The length of a candle's burn time is determined by the type of wax and its size.

TAPER CANDLES

Taper candles come in all different lengths and dimensions. If you're doing a working that requires you to light the candle over the course of several days, consider a longer taper; you can even make a series of marks on the wax, so you know how long to let it burn each day. One of the most popular forms of taper candle is the chime, or spell candle, which is about four inches long and half an inch in diameter. These candles take a few hours to burn and can often be purchased in boxes that include a selection of colors. Because they're so thin, though, it can be a challenge to find a candle holder to fit them properly and safely.

TEA LIGHTS

Tea lights are the most inexpensive and practical candle to use in many spells. They are about an inch and a half in diameter and less than an inch tall, and are often available in multipacks. The average tea light will burn for three to six hours. Consider tea lights for short workings, or for those in which you need multiple candles to represent a variety of concepts or items. Because they're short and typically come in a plastic or metal holder, tea lights aren't usually conducive to dressing with oils or herbs.

PILLAR CANDLES

Like tapers, pillar candles come in a variety of heights and diameters, and sometimes they have multiple wicks. Some of the larger ones with three wicks can get up to a hundred hours of burn time, so if you're doing a working that runs over a period of several days or is boosted regularly, consider a pillar candle. They're freestanding because they have wide bases, so they don't need a candle holder per se, but they should still be placed on a fire-safe surface, like a plate or cauldron.

VOTIVE CANDLES

A votive candle is about two inches tall and about an inch and a half in diameter. A well-made votive will burn for ten to twelve hours, so they're great for spells that run the course of an entire day. Although they're a little more expensive than tea lights, you can often find them in multipacks, and they work nicely for a light dressing of oils and herbs. You can place a votive candle in a small glass jar for safety.

JAR CANDLES

Many people don't like to use jar candles—those that are pre-poured into a glass container—for spellwork because you can't inscribe them or add oil and herbs to the sides. However, you can still decorate the glass jar with paint, markers, or even découpage, so they certainly have their uses. Depending on their size, jar candles can burn for several days before running out of wax. They're often scented, so be sure the fragrance aligns with your magical intent.

BEESWAX, SOY, AND PARAFFIN CANDLES

Many practitioners have a preference when it comes to types of wax. Beeswax is a little more expensive, but it's also usually unscented, other than a sweet natural aroma. It's a harder wax and is eco-friendly. Soy candles burn slowly and are an excellent choice for those who are sensitive to burning wax or who are vegan. Soy can burn unevenly at times, however, and cause your candle to look patchy. Paraffin wax is the least expensive and can hold a great deal of fragrance, but it's also environmentally unfriendly because it's made from a petroleum byproduct.

PREPARING CANDLES FOR USE

As with other magical tools, prepare your candles for use before you get started on a working. You'll want a sacred space where you can perform your spells and rituals; because the space is sacred, you should bring only sacred things into it. It's also important to cleanse, charge, and consecrate your candles before use.

Keep in mind that some spells are designed to be performed at specific times. For instance, many practitioners believe that lunar cycles play a role in a spell's efficacy. Perform spells that are positive or attract things to you during the waxing moon phase, and those that banish or send things away during the waning period. For workings related to self-development and spiritual growth, aim for the time around the full moon.

Days of the week can often play a role in magic as well. Sunday is associated with victory, self-expression, and creativity, whereas spells for healing, wisdom, and intuition are connected with Monday. On Tuesday, workings related to challenges and conflict work best, and Wednesday is connected to communication, jobs, and travel. For Thursday, focus on magic related to success and prosperity, and make Friday the day for fertility and family life. Finally, wrap up the week on Saturday with spells for banishing and protection.

CREATING A SPACE FOR MAGIC

Magic is a sacred activity, so it's crucial to have a special spot for your workings. Not everyone has the ability to have an altar in place all the time, and that's okay. If you can't have a permanent altar, you can still create a space that's dedicated to your magical practice. Even if it's a single bookshelf or the top of a dresser, designate your workspace as a spot for magic and nothing else. Make sure your space is physically as well as metaphysically tidy: Do a regular cleansing by burning sacred herbs or sprinkling consecrated water around the area. Keep your magical tools neatly organized, and if possible, avoid cluttering the space with items that aren't in use. If you have the ability, decorate it with art and other items that make you feel more spiritually grounded and complete.

CLEANSING CANDLES

Like other magical tools, candles pick up the energy of things—or people—they've been in contact with. Cleansing is an important step because it gets rid of all those other residual energies. There are a number of ways to cleanse a candle, and the method isn't important as long as it gets done. Some people like to leave candles outside overnight in the moonlight, whereas others opt to sprinkle them with consecrated water. You might wish to bury your candle in sea salt for twenty-four hours or simply pass it through the smoke of burning sacred herbs. Finally, you might want to try an elemental cleansing, in which the candle is surrounded by symbols of the four elements—earth, air, fire, and water—and blessed. As you cleanse your candle, visualize any lingering negative energy being banished and sent away.

CHARGING CANDLES

Charging is the method by which we imbue an object with positive magical energy. Sometimes called programming or enchanting, it's a way to give the item a magical boost, a bit like charging a battery. As with cleansing, there are a number of different methods, but this simple one works well. Sit at your altar or workstation and hold the candle in your hand. Close your eyes, and envision positive energy flowing into the candle and enveloping it. It may help to visualize that energy in a color that corresponds with your intent: a green glow for abundance, a red one for passion, and so forth. Some people find it helpful to chant, meditate, or otherwise raise energy during this process.

CONSECRATING CANDLES

Finally, consecrating a candle is the process by which we turn it into a truly spiritual tool. Again, there are a variety of methods you can use. You can say a prayer over it, such as *I dedicate this candle to positive magic so it will bring abundance and blessings into my life.* If you work with a particular deity, you can ask them to bless it as well. If you work with sacred oils, anoint the base of the candle with a small drop and state an affirmation of the intended purpose. You may also wish to pass it over symbols of the four elements—a bowl of soil, a feather, another candle's flame, and a glass of consecrated water. Remember that once a candle or any other item is consecrated, it is sacred and should be treated as such.

THE MAGIC OF INTENTION

In the magical community we talk a lot about setting intentions, but what does it actually mean? Consider, for a moment, that intention without action is simply making a wish. And although wishing is great, it doesn't necessarily facilitate transformation. Setting your intention isn't just wishing, it's also making a commitment to yourself that you're going to focus on change and take action to bring those changes about. In other words, intention isn't only the end goal, although that's part of it. It's also about the journey you take to get there, and that journey is how we manifest our dreams.

Many people find that focusing on their purpose helps with setting intentions. For instance, perhaps you want to bring financial abundance into your life, but what for? Is it to pay off a bill? Take your family on a nice vacation? Establish a nest egg? Once you figure out your purpose, it's a lot easier to determine what you want to achieve, why you want to achieve it, and how you can get there.

Allowing yourself to set your intention with purpose and clarity of process will make it much easier to actually do the work. Think of it this way: If you're going on a road trip, you probably know where the end destination will be, but to actually reach it, you've got to look at maps, make sure your car is in working order, figure out where to eat and sleep, get gas along the way, and so on. Once you've determined all those things, your travels will become much more focused.

HOW TO BE INTENTIONAL

So you know you need to focus your intention, but sometimes that's easier said than done. Although everyone sets their intention in a different way, you may find this simple five-step method helpful. By truly putting thought into the process, you'll enhance your spellwork as you become more intentional with your candle magic practice.

MEDITATE ON YOUR MANIFESTATION

Start by giving some careful and logical thought to your magical goal. What do you hope to achieve? It's easy to say, *I am going to be happy*, but that's pretty vague. What are the things that will make you content? How do you personally define happiness? Likewise, if you want abundance, or healing, what do those things look like to you? Take some time to meditate and reflect so you can come up with a truly focused goal for your magic to target.

SET SPECIFIC INTENTIONS

Get specific. Like, really specific. Let's go back to the example of abundance. My definition of abundance might not be the same as yours. For some people, it means the ability to pay their bills without living paycheck to paycheck, or to buy some fancy groceries next time they go shopping. Maybe it's about saving money for a car or paying off a loan so you can be debt free. This moment is where purpose comes into play. What is your specific intention? Make magic, not wish-craft. Use active, present-tense statements, such as *I am wealthy* or *I am debt free*, rather than *I would like to have extra money* or *I don't want to be burdened by debt*.

SET REALISTIC INTENTIONS

It's crucial that your intentions be realistic. The *probability* of something happening is far more relevant than the *possibility*. Going back to our abundance example, attracting enough money to pay your electric bill is pretty realistic, but winning the lottery, although certainly possible, is not probable. The more realistic your intentions, the more likely you'll be to successfully manifest them.

SET ETHICAL INTENTIONS

Everyone has their own set of magical ethics, and it's important to establish boundaries for yourself. If there are things that you'll never do, magically, you should stick with that decision. You may find it helpful to craft a personal statement of ethics to help yourself follow your own guidelines. Make sure your intentions meet these guidelines. In general, most practitioners try to follow ethical standards that avoid doing harm to others; keep in mind, however, that avoiding harm doesn't mean you have to allow others to mistreat you.

ARTICULATE INTENTIONS THROUGH POSITIVITY

When you're setting your intentions, use active, positive language. In fact, you may find it helpful to articulate your intentions in a way that assumes they already have happened or, at the very least, are sure to manifest. Instead of *I wish I were happy*, try *I am happy*. Rather than *I hope I'll find love someday*, consider *I will find love* or *Love is coming into my life*. When you focus your intentions in an active and positive way, making them manifest is the logical resolution.

CHOOSING SPELLS FOR TRANSFORMATION

When you're doing spellwork for self-transformation, you'll likely find that most of your intentions fall into a few key categories: love, protection, healing, prosperity, and happiness. As you're selecting spells to perform, remember that intention not only influences the outcome, but also encourages you to practice with purpose. As you focus more on purpose in your magical life, you'll begin to do so in the mundane, or nonmagical, aspects of your world as well. Practicing magic is transformative not only because of what the magic brings us but also because of what the process *teaches* us.

As a result, it's important to understand the connection between your intention and the spell itself. Think carefully about how you word things. Remember the old chestnut about being careful what you wish for because you just might get it? If you're not mindful of what you're putting out into the universe, you may find yourself with a result that's completely unexpected and yet still in line with what you articulated as an intention.

LOVE

Love spells are perhaps one of the most hotly debated topics in the magical community. Many people feel you should never do a love spell aimed at a specific person because it interferes with the individual's free will. In theory, all magic interferes with *something*, because the entire point of practicing is to change the things we find unsatisfying.

Regardless of how you feel about love spells, you'll probably find that an honest and ethical way to work love magic is to work it upon yourself. Do spellwork that makes you feel more confident and poised. Work up some candle magic that boosts your self-esteem to remind you that you are deserving and worthy of being loved. Craft a working that shows the rest of the world you are attractive and appealing.

PROTECTION

A good magical self-defense system is a valuable thing indeed. Protection magic can be done in a variety of forms and for a number of different purposes. You may want to protect your house, car, or property. Maybe you want to keep yourself and your family safe from physical attack—or perhaps you feel a need to work up some protection from the things we can't see, like spiritual entities or the chaos caused by other magical practitioners.

In addition to active, defensive protection magic, you may find that banishing spells work well for you. Banishing eliminates negative people, things, or energies from your life. If banishing isn't an option, perhaps a binding might serve you better. Binding is the act of preventing someone from doing harm to themselves or other people. Again, determining your intention and purpose will help you craft the right type of working for your situation.

HEALING

When it comes to healing, you can focus your magic on caring for the mind, body, or spirit. By setting specific intentions for healing magic, you will be able to take a holistic approach to bringing about change and transformation. Healing magic can encompass surrounding a sick person with positive energy, reducing stress, or even just focusing on self-care so you can get through a challenging situation without losing control. Target your healing candle magic on yourself or others, depending on need.

Remember, although magic is a useful healing tool, if you or someone you love is in crisis, spellwork is not a substitute for professional medical or mental health care. Seek out the proper treatment you need, and remember there is never any shame in asking for assistance.

PROSPERITY AND ABUNDANCE

Most practitioners in modern magical traditions find prosperity magic works best when spellwork is done from need rather than greed. You might love the idea of inheriting a million bucks, but someone has to die for that to happen. Instead, focus on reducing debt, paying bills, and setting aside money for future expenses. If you work prosperity magic in small chunks, you'll likely find that it's cumulative, and you'll grow your abundance gradually.

Again, keep in mind that abundance means different things to everyone. For many people, it might be financial, but for others, it could be professional success, a loving family life, or a circle of friends that lifts you up rather than pushes you down. Determine how you define abundance, and manifest change and transformation from there.

HAPPINESS AND WELL-BEING

There's a good deal of overlap between healing and happiness. Doing spells for self-improvement and your own well-being isn't selfish. In fact, it's self-enhancing. The more you take care of yourself, the better you'll feel—and when you feel better, you'll share that joy with those who surround you, leading to happier, more loving relationships. It goes full circle, because as your relationships improve, you'll continue to feel good, which you'll share, and so on.

Remember, your happiness and well-being should never be dependent upon the actions or words of others. Changing someone else won't make you happy (and often isn't feasible), but what you can change is how you feel about their behaviors and how you react. By creating a sense of inner happiness, you'll be able to transform yourself into someone with healthy coping skills, fulfilling relationships, and an empowered spirit.

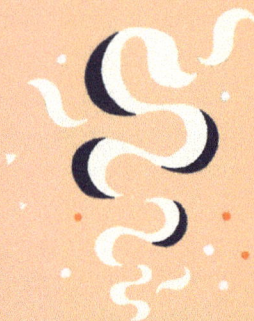

YOU MUST BE THE BEST JUDGE
OF YOUR OWN HAPPINESS.

—JANE AUSTEN

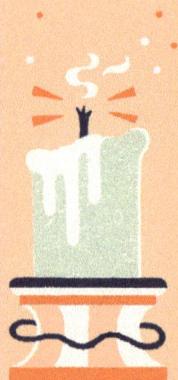

PART 2

PROMPTS FOR PERSONAL REFLECTION AND INTENTION SETTING

Now that we've reviewed some of the fundamentals of candle magic, it's time to start evaluating your intentions and setting goals. What do you hope to achieve with magic? How do you wish to transform your life?

In this section, there is a series of prompts and questions to ask yourself. You may find some uncomfortable, but all of them will remind you that by speaking your truth, you can discover authenticity of purpose. Once you've allowed yourself to be a little bit vulnerable by revealing your intention, you'll be ready to move on to part 3 and start doing the work.

YOUR MAGICAL MISSION STATEMENT: Each of us is a magical being, but everyone is magical in a different way. What makes you magical? What do you hope to achieve with your practice of magic, spellwork, and ritual?

_____

_____

_____

_____

_____

_____

_____

_____

_____

WHERE HAVE YOU BEEN? We're all shaped by our past experiences, regardless of whether they're good or bad. What is one event in your life that profoundly shaped and influenced the person you are today? How did it affect you?

_____

_____

_____

_____

_____

_____

_____

_____

_____

WHERE ARE YOU GOING? Think about your answer to the previous question regarding an event in your past that shaped you. How will that particular situation influence your future and the journey ahead of you in life?

_____

_____

_____

_____

_____

_____

_____

_____

_____

HEAL YOUR HEART: We've all experienced heartache, and it can be devastating. Think about a time your heart hurt. What support do you wish you'd had? What advice or compassion would you offer a friend who's going through the same thing?

_____

_____

_____

_____

_____

_____

_____

_____

PROTECT YOUR SPACE: Your home is a place where you should feel physically, emotionally, and spiritually safe. Imagine you could surround your home with a protective shield, net, or barrier. What would it look like? How would it shelter and protect you?

_____

_____

_____

_____

_____

_____

_____

_____

LIGHT A SACRED FLAME: Candle magic is just one of many forms of magic. What do you hope to achieve with your practice? What does a candle flame symbolize to you, and what draws you to using its transformative power?

_____

_____

_____

_____

_____

_____

_____

_____

KEYS TO SUCCESS: How do you define success—professional, personal, or otherwise? If you could snap your fingers and be successful, what would that entail? Would you view yourself differently?

_____

_____

_____

_____

_____

_____

_____

_____

_____

THE LANGUAGE OF LOVE: In matters of love, many of us want someone whose communication style matches ours. What expressions of love would be most meaningful to you, and how would you express your own feelings?

_____

_____

_____

_____

_____

_____

_____

_____

_____

GOOD VIBRATIONS: Think about the energy you put out into the world. Is a negative mindset keeping you from living a vibrant, magical life? How can you reframe your thoughts in a way that helps you focus on the positive?

FIND YOUR COURAGE: Picture the most fearless person you know. What do you admire about them? Now visualize yourself with those same courageous attributes. What would you try if fear wasn't an obstacle, and what would you do with your new experience?

ADVISE YOUR INNER CHILD: Imagine yourself a child again, with your entire life ahead of you. Write a letter to that child, giving them the advice and wisdom you've collected and what you wish you'd known back then.

_____

_____

_____

_____

_____

_____

_____

_____

_____

BE RADICALLY KIND: It's great to be acknowledged when we do things for others, but what about kindness for its own sake? Do something nice for someone else without telling them. Is your action still meaningful if you don't receive praise afterward?

_____

_____

_____

_____

_____

_____

_____

_____

_____

FIGHT OR FLIGHT: What is your immediate response when encountering conflict? Do you tackle things head-on or escape the situation to avoid it altogether? How can you emotionally or mentally prepare yourself ahead of time so you can face challenges with poise?

_____

_____

_____

_____

_____

_____

_____

_____

_____

BOUNTY AND BLESSINGS: People often mention counting their blessings. Consider three things for which you are truly grateful. Write a thank-you letter to the universe and to those who have brought joy to your world.

_____

_____

_____

_____

_____

_____

_____

_____

_____

FRIENDSHIP CIRCLE: Identifying positive qualities in others can help you find and keep friends, as well as help you *be* a better friend. Write down the traits that matter to you most in a friendship and why they're important.

_____

_____

_____

_____

_____

_____

_____

_____

_____

WHERE DO YOU DRAW THE LINE? Are there certain types of magic you have decided you'll never do? What limits will you set for yourself in your practice? Determine your boundaries and decide what types of magic are ethically off-limits for you and why.

_____

_____

_____

_____

_____

_____

_____

_____

_____

ONE STEP AT A TIME: It's hard to learn unfamiliar concepts. Breaking them down into smaller pieces can make them easier to understand. What are you really struggling to comprehend, and what small steps can you build upon to help conquer the challenge?

_____

_____

_____

_____

_____

_____

_____

_____

_____

MONEY OR HAPPINESS? If you were rich beyond your wildest dreams, would it solve your problems? Would you rather (a) have all the money you need but not be truly happy, or (b) live on a tight budget but be completely content? Why?

_____

_____

_____

_____

_____

_____

_____

_____

_____

FIND YOUR COMFORT ZONE: When and where do you feel most relaxed and at peace? What can you do to carry that feeling with you, even when you're in a situation that makes you anxious and stressed out?

_____

_____

_____

_____

_____

_____

_____

_____

_____

CELEBRATE YOURSELF: Write about something you've done that made you feel strong and confident. What about that event was inspiring and memorable? How can you re-create and celebrate that feeling of pride and self-confidence regularly?

_____

_____

_____

_____

_____

_____

_____

_____

_____

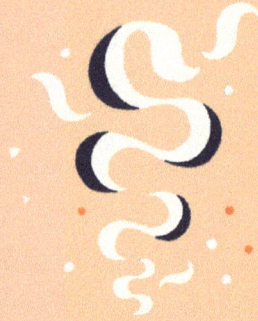

THE UNIVERSE IS FULL OF MAGICAL
THINGS PATIENTLY WAITING FOR
OUR WITS TO GROW SHARPER.

—EDEN PHILLPOTTS

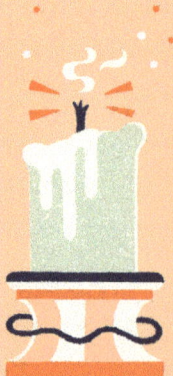

PART 3

PRACTICE YOUR MAGIC AND RECORD YOUR PROGRESS

Now that you've had an opportunity to reflect upon where you've been and where you want to go, it's time to make some magic! Before you begin, consider the energy you plan to release into the world. If the energy you put out is negative, plan to be held accountable. Likewise, surrounding yourself with positive energy—and magic—can bring good things back to you.

In this section, you'll encounter 15 candle magic spells, focusing on affection and attraction, protection, healing, prosperity and abundance, and happiness and well-being. Don't limit yourself to the spells found here, though. Instead, use them as guidelines for basic spell construction, and take time to answer the questions after each working. Doing so will give you an opportunity to reflect on your results, learn from what you've done, and plan for next time.

Note that when you extinguish a candle used for magical purposes, unless the spell specifically calls for it, don't blow it out. Use a snuffer or other tool instead.

PATIENTLY WAITING FOR YOUR SPELL

Despite what you've probably seen on television, spellwork isn't a quick fix. If instant gratification is what you're looking for, magic might not be your jam. Like anything else worth having, magical results take not only work but also *time*. In general, most practitioners agree that if the spell worked, you'll start seeing results within 28 days, or one lunar cycle. Does that mean the working will be completely finished in a month? Not necessarily, but it does mean that if your magic manifests successfully, that period is when you'll start to see hints that it's taking effect.

This waiting period is another reason it's valuable to write things down. Watch for subtle differences in your world after a spell is cast. Sometimes results unfold right before our eyes, and we don't even realize it! Learn to be patient.

SPELLS FOR ATTRACTION AND AFFECTION

Many people feel it's unethical to do attraction spells aimed at a specific person. However, it's acceptable to do magical workings that help you present yourself in a way that draws people to you. The spells in this section have been created to attract new relationships, encourage affection, and boost your appeal to those with whom you want to cultivate healthy, caring relationships. Don't consider them "love spells"; instead, think of them in terms of self-love workings, designed in a way that can bring you and someone special together.

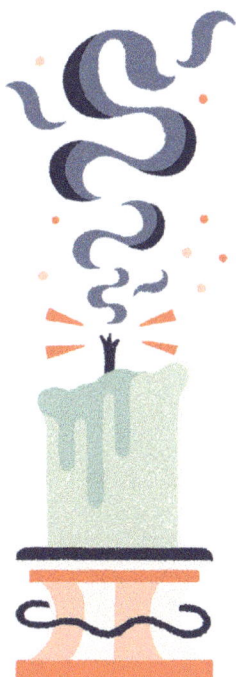

THE LANGUAGE OF LOVE

We each speak our own language in matters of love—perhaps you express yourself with words, physical actions, giving gifts, or cooking a meal. Think about your love communication style. What meaningful things can your partner say or do to show affection? While doing this working, think about your ideal partner bringing these words or actions to life. Try to perform this spell on a Friday, a day associated with many goddesses of love.

INGREDIENTS

Scissors

Red paper

A permanent marker

A red jar candle

With the scissors, cut out a paper heart, and on it, use the marker to write examples of loving words or actions you'd like to see in a potential partner. Place the candle on top of the heart and light it. Watch the flame, and say,

> *My heart speaks to yours, and yours to mine. I speak words of love and hear yours in return. I give love and receive your love in return.*

As you speak, visualize these romantic messages coming to fruition.

Allow the candle to burn for three hours, and then extinguish it. Keep the candle in a place where you'd like to spend time with your partner. Repeat as needed on Fridays until the candle has burned away.

Date and Time of Spell: _____

Intention and Purpose: _____

How Did You Feel Afterward? _____

Reflect on Changes: _____

_____

Additional Notes: _____

_____

_____

_____

_____

_____

_____

_____

_____

_____

_____

_____

_____

_____

_____

_____

_____

BEACON OF FRIENDSHIP

Not everyone needs or wants romance—platonic loving relationships are equally valuable, if you find the right people. This simple working creates a beacon of light to draw new friends and form happy, healthy, positive relationships. Do this spell during the waxing moon phase, associated with attraction magic; perform the working outside if possible.

INGREDIENTS

An inscribing tool
A pink pillar candle
A candle holder

9 yellow rose petals, fresh
  or dried

Inscribe the words *love*, *loyalty*, and *trust* around the candle. Place the candle in a fire-safe holder and surround it with the rose petals. Light the candle and take some time to focus on the flame itself. Visualize it as a beacon in the darkness, inviting people toward you. Say,

I value love, I value loyalty, I value trust. These are the qualities I seek in new friends. Let those who exhibit these traits recognize them in me, as I open myself to forging new relationships. May only those who are loving, loyal, and trustworthy enter my circle.

Continue envisioning new friends, attracted to your beacon, who will lift you up. Imagine the ways you can enrich each other's lives. When you begin to feel restless or bored, extinguish the candle. Dispose of the candle and the rose petals somewhere near your home, either by burying them or hiding them in a spot where they will be undisturbed.

Date and Time of Spell: _____

Intention and Purpose: _____

How Did You Feel Afterward? _____

Reflect on Changes: _____

_____

Additional Notes: _____

_____

_____

_____

_____

_____

_____

_____

_____

_____

_____

_____

_____

_____

_____

_____

_____

HAPPY FAMILY FLAME SPELL

Sometimes a little magic can go a long way to boost love between family members. Strengthen your family ties with a spell to bring you closer together, creating stability and security. Do this working on a Wednesday, a day tied to matters of communication.

INGREDIENTS

Soil, sand, or stones from a place meaningful to your family

A wide fire-safe dish

A bay leaf

A pink votive candle for each family member

Place a layer of soil, sand, or stones in the bottom of the dish. Set the bay leaf, associated with communication, on top of the layer. Finally, place the candles on top of the bay leaf, clustering them close together, and as you put each candle in the dish, assign it the name of one family member. Add some more soil, sand, or stones around the candles so they sit securely.

Light the candles, and with each one, say,

[Name], I love you and am so glad you are part of my family. With this flame, may our love burn bright, bringing us joy, love, stability, and hope. Once all the candles are lit, say, *A single candle burns bright, but a group burns brighter. We are strong individually but stronger together. May our family's light always shine.*

Reflect on the actions you need to take to help your family rediscover love. Allow the candles to burn out on their own, then bury them someplace close to home.

Date and Time of Spell: _____

Intention and Purpose: _____

How Did You Feel Afterward? _____

Reflect on Changes: _____

_____

Additional Notes: _____

_____

_____

_____

_____

_____

_____

_____

_____

_____

_____

_____

_____

_____

_____

_____

_____

_____

REFLECT ON YOUR PROGRESS

You've had an opportunity to do candle magic for different types of love. How do you feel about using magic to draw affection into your life? What mundane, or nonmagical, actions will you take in tandem with your spellwork to attract love?

_____

_____

_____

_____

_____

_____

_____

_____

_____

_____

_____

_____

_____

_____

_____

_____

_____

_____

_____

_____

SPELLS FOR PROTECTION

Candles can be used effectively for protection magic, which can keep your home and family physically safe, shield you from those who would speak ill of you, or purge negative energy from your space. Remember, mundane actions can often be taken in tandem with spellwork—for instance, if you're worried about break-ins at your home, in addition to casting a spell, be sure to keep doors and windows locked. Use common sense. It's one of the most important ingredients in any magical working.

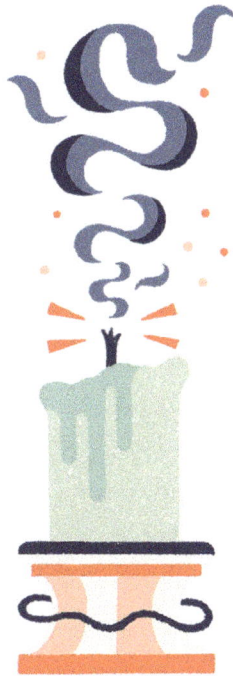

MAGICAL PURIFICATION CANDLE

In addition to keeping our space physically tidy, it's a good idea to do some metaphysical cleansing now and again. Do this working to purify your sacred space and keep negative energy, psychic entities, or plain old bad vibes from getting in. To dress the candle, use a lightweight unscented oil. Do this spell over seven consecutive nights.

INGREDIENTS

An inscribing tool
A white pillar candle
Unscented oil

Any purification herb—such as mugwort, rosemary, mullein, or goldenrod— ground finely

Using your inscribing tool, mark lines on the candle to divide it into seven equal segments. With a small brush or piece of cotton, apply a thin layer of oil around the candle, working from the top to the middle and then from the base to the middle. Roll the oiled candle in the herb, covering it with a fine layer.

Light the candle, saying,

I purify this space, I cleanse this space, I consecrate this space. No evil shall enter, no negativity shall enter, no harm shall enter. This space is pure, this space is cleansed, this place is sacred.

Let the candle burn down to the first score line and then extinguish it. Repeat for seven consecutive nights, until the candle is gone.

Date and Time of Spell: _____

Intention and Purpose: _____

How Did You Feel Afterward? _____

Reflect on Changes: _____

_____

Additional Notes: _____

_____

_____

_____

_____

_____

_____

_____

_____

_____

_____

_____

_____

_____

_____

_____

_____

HOME SWEET HOME PROTECTION SPELL

Whether you live in a small city apartment, a sprawling suburban house, or anything in between, your home is your castle. In addition to taking nonmagical precautions, do this simple protection spell to keep you and your family safe from those who might cause mischief. Do this working at night, during the full moon.

INGREDIENTS

One yellow votive candle for each exterior door of your home

One hematite stone for each window

Iron nails, pins, or spikes

Starting with the front entrance and working around the inside perimeter of your home, place a candle at each door, a hematite stone at each window, and an iron nail in each outer corner. Once they're in position, light the candle at the front door, and say,

My home is my castle, safe, secure, and sound. Let no trouble-makers ever come around.

Walk around your house, stopping to repeat these words at each window, door, and corner, and lighting each candle as you reach it. Visualize the light from the candles enveloping your home in a protective yellow glow. When you return to the front entrance, stop and envision that yellow glow expanding, surrounding the outside of your home, to keep you and your loved ones safe.

Allow the candles to burn for an hour, and then keep them near your doors in case you need to repeat the working in the future.

Date and Time of Spell: _____

Intention and Purpose: _____

How Did You Feel Afterward? _____

Reflect on Changes: _____

_____

Additional Notes: _____

_____

_____

_____

_____

_____

_____

_____

_____

_____

_____

_____

_____

_____

_____

_____

_____

SHUT THE HECK UP CANDLE

If you know someone who can't keep their opinions of you out of their mouth—or who likes to gossip, tell lies, or spread information that isn't their business—this spell is for you. To dress the candle, use a lightweight unscented oil, like grapeseed or safflower, and dried dill, which is associated with silence. Use a mortar and pestle or another grinding tool to crush the herb.

INGREDIENTS

An inscribing tool

A black candle

Unscented oil

Dried dill, ground finely

Inscribe the name of your problem person on the candle. Using a small brush or piece of cotton, apply a thin layer of oil around the candle, moving away from you. Roll the oiled candle in the dill, so the outside is covered in a fine coating of dried herb.

Light the candle, and visualize the person who's been speaking about you. Say,

[Name], your words have no power. Your words mean nothing. Your words about me will no longer be heard. They will fall upon deaf ears, and my name will no longer come from your mouth. Your words have no power at all. You will be silent.

As you do so, envision the person's words about you floating away into nothingness, so they no longer exist. Allow the candle to burn out on its own, and then take it someplace far from your home to dispose of it.

Date and Time of Spell: _____

Intention and Purpose: _____

How Did You Feel Afterward? _____

Reflect on Changes: _____

_____

Additional Notes: _____

_____

_____

_____

_____

_____

_____

_____

_____

_____

_____

_____

_____

_____

_____

_____

_____

REFLECT ON YOUR PROGRESS

You've now done candle magic for various kinds of protection. What other applications can you think of for protection magic? Are there other items with protective properties you can combine with candle magic?

_____

_____

_____

_____

_____

_____

_____

_____

_____

_____

_____

_____

_____

_____

_____

_____

_____

_____

SPELLS FOR HEALING

Healing magic is found all over the world. In a magical context, candles can help bring about physical wellness, emotional benefits, and overall good feelings. Many people like to use scented candles for healing magic because of the benefits of aromatherapy, but you don't have to unless you feel called to do so.

Additionally, remember that magical workings are no substitute for treatment by a medical or mental health professional. If you need it, seek out help from those qualified to give it. Your emotional and physical well-being is important, so don't be afraid to request support.

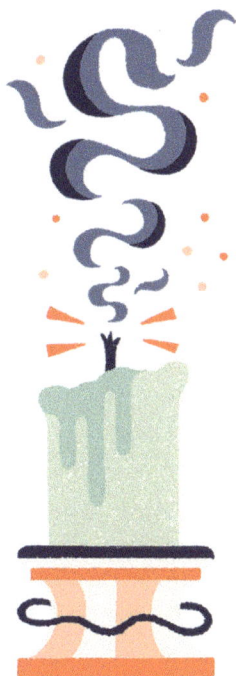

WELLNESS AND HEALING CANDLE BATH

Humans are holistic creatures. When we feel poorly physically, emotionally, or spiritually, everything gets thrown off-kilter. Although it's important to take good physical and mental care of ourselves, every once in a while, we just need a boost. Do this working at the end of your day, when you can relax and not be disturbed.

INGREDIENTS

Healing herbs such as chamomile, echinacea, lavender, rosemary, basil, feverfew, etc.

A small cloth drawstring bag
A bathtub
3 light blue candles

Place the herbs in the drawstring bag, pulling it closed. Hang the bag over your tub's water faucet and fill the bath with warm water, allowing it to course over the herbs. Place the candles along the edge of the tub and light them. Get into the bath, and soak in the warm herb-scented water. Focus on the first candle, and say,

I draw healing magic from this flame, so that I can be my best physical self. Study the flame of the second, saying, *I draw healing magic from this flame, so I can be my best emotional self.* Finally, gaze upon the last one, and say, *I draw healing magic from this flame, so that I can be my best spiritual self.*

Sit in the tub, visualizing the healing energy of the three flames surrounding you. When the water has cooled off, get out of the tub and extinguish the candles. Let the water drain, taking away with it anything that has you feeling unwell.

Date and Time of Spell: _____

Intention and Purpose: _____

How Did You Feel Afterward? _____

Reflect on Changes: _____

_____

Additional Notes: _____

_____

_____

_____

_____

_____

_____

_____

_____

_____

_____

_____

_____

_____

_____

_____

_____

PET HEALING CANDLE

It's so hard when our pets feel poorly. They're part of our families, and often they don't understand what's going on. If you've got a beloved pet who's unwell, do this simple spell to help send them some healing energy. Remember, candle magic should never replace proper care; if your pet needs veterinary treatment, get them to a professional for help. This spell can be done whenever it is needed. If possible, invite your pet to join you as you perform the working.

INGREDIENTS

A photo of your pet
An amethyst crystal

A brown candle
Lavender essential oil

Lay the photo of your pet on your workspace or altar and place the amethyst on top. Dress the candle by anointing it with the lavender oil, using a small brush or piece of cotton. Light the candle and place it on top of the photo beside the amethyst. As your candle burns, envision the healing energy flowing through the candle and the healing power of the amethyst covering your pet, bringing them relief from pain and discomfort.

While you watch the flame, say,

My beloved [pet's name], you are my family, you are my heart. I send healing energy to you, so you will not hurt, you will not suffer, and so you may recover.

If your pet allows you to touch them, visualize that healing energy flowing into them as you touch their fur or skin. Extinguish the candle and save it so you can repeat as needed.

Date and Time of Spell: _____

Intention and Purpose: _____

How Did You Feel Afterward? _____

Reflect on Changes: _____

_____

Additional Notes: _____

_____

_____

_____

_____

_____

_____

_____

_____

_____

_____

_____

_____

_____

_____

_____

_____

THREE-DAY HEALING SPELL

Call healing into your life when you just can't handle all the nonsense life is throwing at you. The dark blue candle is associated with vulnerability. Perform this spell over three nights, beginning the evening before the full moon and ending the night after.

INGREDIENTS

Your favorite relaxation incense, enough for three nights

A dark blue pillar candle

On the first night, light the incense, allowing the fragrance to relax you. Close your eyes and breathe deeply, taking in its magical aroma. Light the candle. Say,

This night, as the moon waxes, I draw to me healing, tranquility, and strength. I attract these things into my life.

Allow the candle to burn down a third of the way and then extinguish it.

The second night, light your incense, and then light the candle, saying,

This night, as the moon is full, I celebrate my intuition, my wisdom, and my power. I honor these things in myself.

Let the candle burn down and extinguish it when only a third remains.

On the final night, after you've lit the incense and the candle, say,

This night, as the moon begins to wane, I send away fear, pain, stress, and strife. I banish these things from my life.

Let the last third of the candle burn out on its own.

Date and Time of Spell: _____

Intention and Purpose: _____

How Did You Feel Afterward? _____

Reflect on Changes: _____

_____

Additional Notes: _____

_____

_____

_____

_____

_____

_____

_____

_____

_____

_____

_____

_____

_____

_____

_____

_____

REFLECT ON YOUR PROGRESS

Now that you've done some candle magic for healing, how do you feel? Are you beginning to see improvements? Is there someone in your life you can help by offering healing magic on their behalf, if they give permission?

_____

_____

_____

_____

_____

_____

_____

_____

_____

_____

_____

_____

_____

_____

_____

_____

_____

_____

_____

_____

_____

SPELLS FOR PROSPERITY AND ABUNDANCE

One of the common misconceptions about prosperity and abundance spells is that you can do things like win the lottery just by snapping your fingers. Prosperity spells work on a number of different levels, and the key is to remember that sometimes those levels offer opportunities rather than instant payoffs. If you do a prosperity spell and then your boss offers you a chance to work overtime and earn time and a half—well, that's an opportunity. Money earned from work spends just as well as money handed to you.

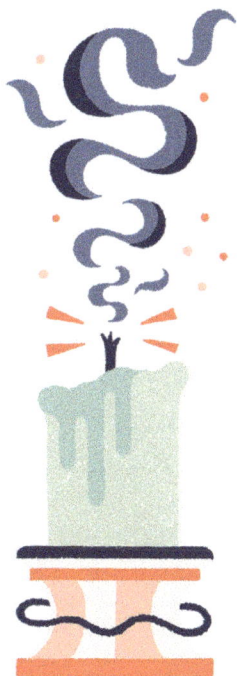

NEED, NOT GREED, SPELL

If you're not obsessed with winning the lottery, an approach of working from need rather than greed will do nicely. For this spell, you'll need unscented oil such as grapeseed or jojoba as a base, and two essential oils known for attracting prosperity. Do this working during the waxing moon phase.

INGREDIENTS

An inscribing tool

A green candle

A small bowl

2 tablespoons unscented oil

2 drops each cinnamon and
   patchouli essential oils

Use the inscribing tool to carve money symbols into the candle. For most people, it's dollar signs, but use whatever resonates most for you. In the bowl, blend the oils together, and then use this mixture to dress your candle with a small brush or piece of cloth, working toward yourself.

Light the candle and say,

I attract money into my life and money into my home. I call money to me for a purpose and will use it responsibly. Money is a blessing, and I welcome opportunities for abundance in my life.

Allow the candle to burn out on its own until there is nothing left.

Date and Time of Spell: _____

Intention and Purpose: _____

How Did You Feel Afterward? _____

Reflect on Changes: _____

_____

Additional Notes: _____

_____

_____

_____

_____

_____

_____

_____

_____

_____

_____

_____

_____

_____

_____

_____

_____

_____

SPELL FOR SMART MONEY MANAGEMENT

If you're struggling financially, this spell can help banish unwanted expenses as you become a better money manager. Write out a detailed monthly household budget prior to doing this working. Try to do it on a Wednesday or Thursday.

INGREDIENTS

A piece of paper

A pen

A gold candle

A fire-safe dish

Draw a line down the center of the paper. On one side of the line, list every source of income your household has during the month. On the other, write down every expense you have. Add them up and look at the differences in the totals. Would you like one to be higher and one to decrease? Tear the paper in half, along the line. Place the income half on your workstation and set the candle on top of it. Light the candle, and visualize money and abundance flowing down to your list of income sources. Say,

Money, I call you to me, following a path into my home.

Light the half of the paper with your debt in the candle's flame. Drop it in the fire-safe dish, and as it burns, say,

Debt, I send you away from me, following a path away from my home.

Allow the candle to burn out on its own. Follow your budget wisely, and when you have to make financial decisions, determine whether you want debt or income.

Date and Time of Spell: _____

Intention and Purpose: _____

How Did You Feel Afterward? _____

Reflect on Changes: _____

_____

Additional Notes: _____

_____

_____

_____

_____

_____

_____

_____

_____

_____

_____

_____

_____

_____

_____

_____

ABUNDANCE GRATITUDE CANDLE

Abundance isn't just about money. Many people believe that gratitude attracts more bounty. What are you thankful to already have? What do you want to attract? This spell uses crystals associated with prosperity and blessings. If possible, do this working on a Sunday, a day associated with action and change.

INGREDIENTS

Images or photos that represent abundance to you

A paintbrush and clear or white glue

A white jar candle

A crystal associated with abundance, such as pyrite or citrine

Cut out photos or pictures that symbolize abundance. Use the brush and glue to découpage them onto the outside of the jar. As you work, think about the blessings you already have in your life, the things for which you are already grateful. Once your images are in place, light the candle. Place the crystal beside it.

Visualize the abundant life you want. Speak it out loud, if you wish, enumerating everything you hope to achieve and obtain. As you do, remember that when you eventually get what you want, it's important to give thanks for those things as well. Envision yourself expressing gratitude in the future when your goals are realized. Allow the candle to burn itself out. Carry the crystal in your pocket as a talisman to attract abundance.

Date and Time of Spell: _____

Intention and Purpose: _____

How Did You Feel Afterward? _____

Reflect on Changes: _____

_____

Additional Notes: _____

_____

_____

_____

_____

_____

_____

_____

_____

_____

_____

_____

_____

_____

_____

_____

_____

REFLECT ON YOUR PROGRESS

Now that you've done some prosperity magic, has it changed your perception of what abundance actually means to you? Are there nonfinancial ways prosperity spells could be beneficial in your life?

_____

_____

_____

_____

_____

_____

_____

_____

_____

_____

_____

_____

_____

_____

_____

_____

_____

_____

_____

_____

_____

SPELLS FOR HAPPINESS AND WELL-BEING

Everyone has a different definition of what it means to be happy. However you describe it, finding your happy is an empowering and self-fulfilling action—the happier you are, the more joy you are likely to attract. By clearing out the things that don't make you content, you open up more space for the things that bring you pleasure and delight.

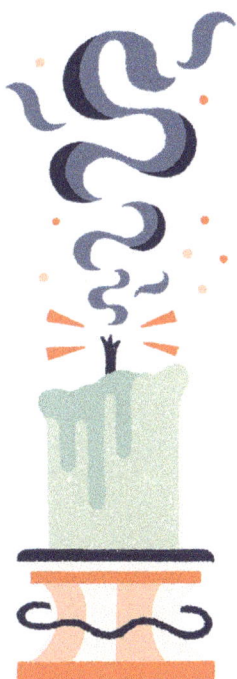

STRESS BUSTER CANDLE

Life is busy, and we all know it! If you're overscheduled, overworked, and underappreciated, it's often hard to find joy in the small things. Use this spell to bust the stress out of your life so you can find some peace, keep calm, and carry on. Do this working outside in the morning, ideally at sunrise, before you've tackled your chaotic day. If it helps you focus, put on some of your favorite relaxing music or sounds in the background.

INGREDIENTS

A light blue candle

Fresh sprigs of your favorite
  calming herb

A tumbled rose quartz stone

Sit on the ground, light the candle, and focus on the flame. Hold the sprigs of the herb in your dominant hand and take a few moments to inhale their scent. Breathe in and out quietly, taking in their aroma and watching the candle flicker. Hold the rose quartz in your other hand, feeling the smooth sides, the edges, every facet of the stone.

Visualize stress traveling downward, out of your body and into the soil. Push it down, and as it empties from your mind, see it being replaced with the tranquil scent of the herbs, the cool calmness of the stone, and the powerful, healing energy of the flame. When you feel yourself getting restless, extinguish the candle, but keep it so you can repeat this spell as needed. Carry the stone in your pocket, and if you feel yourself getting stressed out, rub your fingers over it as a reminder of how it feels to be calm.

Date and Time of Spell: _____

Intention and Purpose: _____

How Did You Feel Afterward? _____

Reflect on Changes: _____

_____

Additional Notes: _____

_____

_____

_____

_____

_____

_____

_____

_____

_____

_____

_____

_____

_____

_____

_____

_____

PERSONAL POWER BOOSTER SPELL

Even when life is looking up, sometimes we just get down. Giving your personal power a boost can work wonders. If you feel confident and strong, you can face the challenges you might have once avoided. Try to do this working on a Sunday, which is associated with beauty, self-expression, and victory.

INGREDIENTS

A bunch of your favorite flowers

12 white tea light candles

A purple candle (or any other color you view as a power color)

A mirror

Sit on the floor and, working in a clockwise direction, arrange the flowers in a circle around yourself. Place the tea lights around you, like numbers on a clock, inside the circle of flowers. Place the purple candle in front of you and light it. Focus on its flame, visualizing your personal power growing. Light the tea light at the one o'clock position, look in the mirror, and say,

I am strong, I am confident, I am powerful, I can face any obstacle.

Light the candle in the two o'clock spot, and repeat this phrase, but do it twice. At three o'clock, repeat it three times, and so on, until you repeat it twelve times at the final tea light.

When all 12 tea lights are lit, take some time to feel the energy in your circle. Sense your power growing. Absorb it, revel in it, celebrate it. When the tea lights have burned out, extinguish the purple candle, and keep it in a place of honor where you can relight it as needed.

Date and Time of Spell: _____

Intention and Purpose: _____

How Did You Feel Afterward? _____

Reflect on Changes: _____

_____

Additional Notes: _____

_____

_____

_____

_____

_____

_____

_____

_____

_____

_____

_____

_____

_____

_____

_____

_____

HAPPINESS BOWL RITUAL

Welcoming happiness and well-being into your life doesn't come naturally for most people. Instead, it's a habit we have to cultivate with repeated actions. By keeping a bowl full of tangible reminders of our joy, we can get into the habit of celebrating life's successes. Do this spell anytime, and repeat it regularly as needed.

INGREDIENTS

A yellow candle
A ceramic or stone bowl
Paper and pen

Tumbled stones or crystals
that make you happy

Place the candle in the bowl and light it. Tear the paper into small pieces, and on each one, write down one thing that makes you happy. Fill up as many pieces as you can! Write things like *my dog* or *hockey games* or *girls' night out*. Whatever brings you joy, articulate it. Put each piece of paper into the bowl, surrounding the candle, and place stones or crystals on top of the paper to hold it in place. As you do, say,

> *This is my joy, this is my happiness, this is my reminder of the good things in life.*

Take some time to meditate on your many blessings. Extinguish the candle.

Every few days, light the candle again and add another piece of paper to the bowl with something that has made you smile, allowing your joy to accumulate over time. If you're having a rough day, think about the words already in the bowl, as a reminder of the good.

Date and Time of Spell: _____

Intention and Purpose: _____

How Did You Feel Afterward? _____

Reflect on Changes: _____

_____

Additional Notes: _____

_____

_____

_____

_____

_____

_____

_____

_____

_____

_____

_____

_____

_____

_____

_____

_____

_____

_____

REFLECT ON YOUR PROGRESS

Now that you've worked some candle magic to help boost your own happiness, how will it benefit you? Do you see the world differently when you're happy? How can you spread joy and be a beacon of light to others?

_____

_____

_____

_____

_____

_____

_____

_____

_____

_____

_____

_____

_____

_____

_____

_____

_____

_____

_____

_____

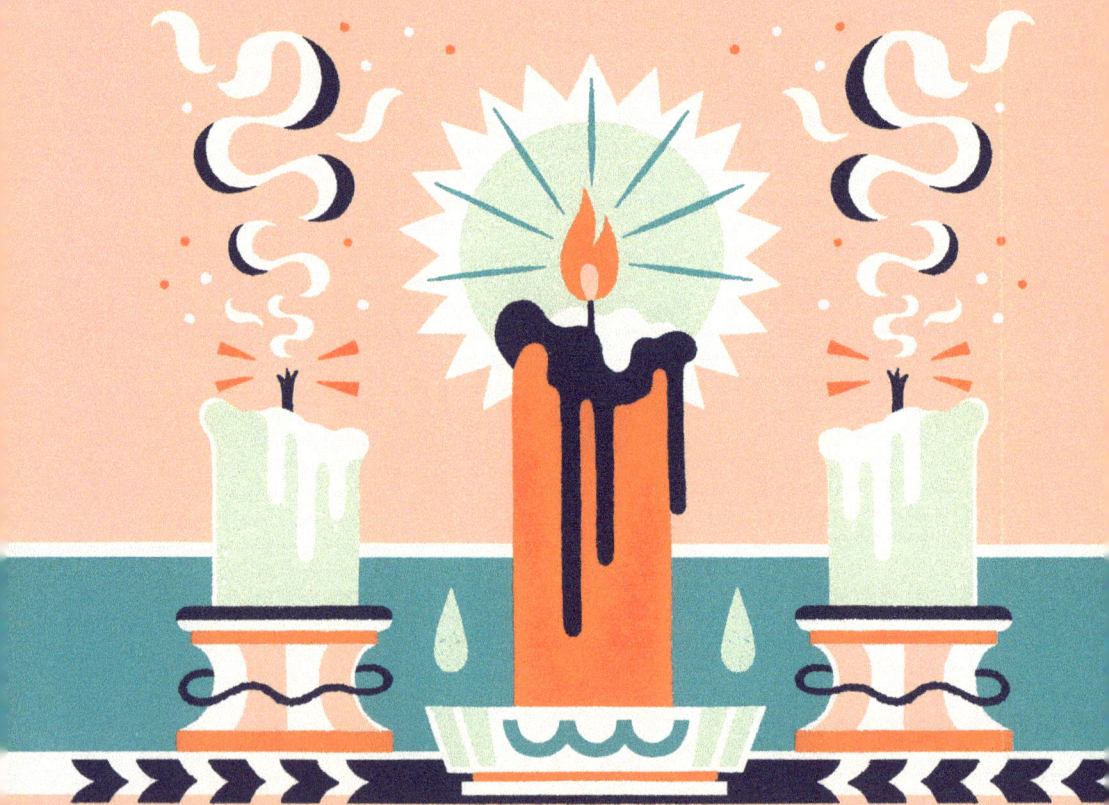

A FINAL WORD

You've made it! Although you might not have done all the spells or answered all the journal prompts—or maybe you did, but the results weren't quite what you expected—you got all the way to the end of this handbook! So now that you have a better understanding of candle magic and how it works, what will you do with it?

Like other forms of magic, candle spells aren't an immediate fix for your problems. They're not one-size-fits-all, and they certainly aren't a substitute for mundane intervention when it's needed. However, they *can* be used effectively as a tool and as a companion to your nonmagical efforts.

When you focus on your intention and your purpose, manifesting change is the next logical occurrence. The flame of a candle can create entire worlds. It can draw and attract abundance, healing, and even love into your life. Fire can also destroy: it's an instrument to banish that which doesn't serve you or to eliminate what brings you down rather than lifts you up. In other words, candle magic is as effective as you choose to make it, in whatever manner you decide to use it.

How will you use candle magic to bring about transformation in your life? What magic can you do to change the things that don't satisfy you? Where will your magical path lead you in the future?

As you're working your magic, take time to pause and reflect, not only on where you've been, but also on where you're going as you move forward. Ask yourself questions, then answer them (even the ones that hurt or are uncomfortable). Getting to know yourself authentically, in a way that is honest and a little bit vulnerable, is the best way to determine the path and eventual outcome of your magic.

And once you've allowed yourself that simple gift, you can change your entire world with a single spark.

RESOURCES

Here are some great books to add to your candle magic collection, suggestions for places to buy candles, and resources for candle-making supplies if you'd like to craft your own.

Buckland, Raymond. *Practical Candleburning Rituals: Spells and Rituals for Every Purpose.* Llewellyn Worldwide, 1982.
This simple handbook includes a number of spells and rituals that can be performed by anyone, regardless of magical experience.

Churchill, Alexandra. "An Introductory Guide to Candle Making." MarthaStewart.com, January 15, 2021. marthastewart.com /8046367/how-to-make-candles.
Instructions for the beginner candle maker, complete with a list of tools and supplies.

Dylan, Mystic. *Candle Magic for Beginners: Spells for Prosperity, Love, Abundance, and More.* Rockridge Press, 2020.
Learn the basics of candle magic, from selecting your candle to preparing your altar for spellwork and rituals.

Pamita, Madame. *The Book of Candle Magic: Candle Spell Secrets to Change Your Life.* Weiser Books, 2020.
Practice the transformational art of candle magic using easy-to-follow rituals, learn to use candles for divination, and make your own candles.

Walker, Tashay. *Candle Magic: The Basics.* Envision Publishing, 2021.
Learn to manifest your goals by taking control of your life through the power of a candle's flame.

Where to Buy Candles

- Your local witchy or metaphysical store

- Vendors in your area—check farmers' markets, gift shops, or locally owned candle stores

- Online retailers such as AzureGreen.com, PracticalMagicStore.com, or TheConjure.com

- Discount stores

REFERENCES

BBC News. "Evidence of 'Earliest Fire Use.'" BBC.com, April 3, 2012. www.bbc.com/news/science-environment-17598738.

Buckland, Raymond. *Buckland's Complete Book of Witchcraft.* Llewellyn, 1986.

Cunningham, Scott. *Encyclopedia of Magical Herbs.* Llewellyn, 1985.

National Candle Association. "History." Candles.org. candles.org /history/.

O'Dea, W. T. "Artificial Lighting Prior to 1800 and Its Social Effects." *Folklore* 62, no. 2 (1951): 312–24. jstor.org/stable/1257599.

Robins, F. W. "The Lamps of Ancient Egypt." *Journal of Egyptian Archaeology* 25, no. 2 (1939): 184–87. doi.org/10.2307/3854653.

Sayer, Karen, and Maryse Helbert. "Illuminating Women: The Case of Candles in the English Home, 1815–1900." *RCC Perspectives* 1 (2020): 30–35. jstor.org/stable/26937550.

Teske, Robert T. "Votive Offerings and the Belief System of Greek-Philadelphians." *Western Folklore* 44, no. 3 (1985): 208–24. doi.org/10.2307/1499836.

Wigington, Patti. *Witchcraft for Healing.* Rockridge Press, 2020.

INDEX

ACKNOWLEDGMENTS

This book wouldn't have been possible without the love and support of the people who put up with my nonsense while I map out an entire manuscript. So much gratitude to my witchy community, my writer friends, and most of all, Caitlin, Zac, and Bree, who know that even when I'm on a deadline, I'll step away from my laptop at a moment's notice just to hear their voices.

ABOUT THE AUTHOR

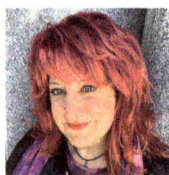

PATTI WIGINGTON has been a practicing witch since 1987, and she works as an educator and workshop facilitator in her local pagan community. She served as the editor of the paganism and Wicca pages at LearnReligions.com (formerly About.com) from 2007 to 2020, and her work has appeared in many pagan magazines, anthologies, and websites. She is licensed pagan clergy and is the founder of Clan of the Stone Circle, a Celtic pagan tradition.

Patti has a BA in history from Ohio University and is the author of several books on modern witchcraft, including *The Good Witch's Daily Spell Book*, *Wicca Practical Magic*, *The Daily Spell Journal*, *Herb Magic*, *Badass Ancestors*, *Witchcraft for Healing*, and *Wicca Journal for Beginners*. She lives in a magical cottage in the woods of southeastern Ohio, where she shares her home with books, art, plants, several dozen tarot decks, and a very large dog. You can find her online at PattiWigington.com or facebook.com/AboutPaganism.

www.ingramcontent.com/pod-product-compliance
Lightning Source LLC
Chambersburg PA
CBHW042047050426
42452CB00019BA/2964